BDSM: The Ultimate Handbook for the Dom and Sub. Training for Pleasure

Introduction

Maybe you've picked up this book because you keep hearing about BDSM through "Fifty Shades of Gray." When it comes to sexual exploration, it's a topic that's hot, but also something that is taboo to talk about. One of the most popular forms of sexual exploration is BDSM.

The problem however, is that BDSM often isn't depicted in the correct manner. Remember when Anna says the safe word in 50 shades and Christian just continues? Yeah, that's not BDSM. BDSM is all about trust, consent, and making the other person feel good.

But why is it so popular? Why do people do it? With some subsections of it including asphyxiation, hair pulling, spankings, and even bondage, it might seem like something you just may not like. But, here is the thing, BDSM is much more than that. You don't go right into hardplay immediately. You start off small. We are going to go over all of the different things you can do when it comes to BDSM, but also give you a couple of important beginner ones to try.

But, there are a few things you must remember before you begin on this journey. Read on and find out all about BDSM, what it entails, and also some important tips, cautions, and tricks to give your partner pleasure.

So, what is BDSM? You may be asking yourself this question after reading 50 Shades, or seeing 50 Shades Freed in theaters. You begin to wonder if it's anything like what Christian Grey did to Anna. The truth is, it's not, and this form does teeter way closer to the level of abuse. But what exactly is it? Why is it something that's considered "pleasurable" for another person? After all, I may seem like something that you shouldn't do, since it does involve hurting another person. Why hurt someone? Why relinquish control? Well, read on, and we'll discuss what it is, and why it matters.

What is BDSM?

BDSM by definition, in the most basic, unadulterated form, is bondage and discipline/dominance and submission or sado-masochism. What that means is that it's an umbrella term that has underneath it any sexual act or mindset that involves two things and they are:

- Dominating
- Relinquishing control

Now, it might seem weird that BDSM is just that after all, why would people relinquish control in the bedroom? The answer is that it can actually be super liberating, and in the long run, if you engage in it, will turn you on in quite a different way compared to other forms of sex.

You've probably looked up BDSM, and you've seen those girls strapped to something tight, and you cringe maybe at the guy smacking her, since you can hear the sounds echoing the truth as well is, that BDSM is actually a very umbrella term, meaning that yes, it involves that, but it also involves having your partner refer to you as sir or madam. It can be a wide variety of things, and it's something that you have to realize, is actually something that has different standards.

You might see the media representation of this as something silly and seedy, or taboo in a sense. However, with new liberation in sexual freedom, the rise of women wanting to take more control of their bodies, and the exploration of sexuality, this type of sexual endeavor is something that many have started to come in contact with, and one that's interested many.

Why enjoy this?

So, what makes this so great? Well, it can create a trusting bond between the woman and the man, unlike anything that's been experienced before. It creates a whole new mindset in women sometimes, since it allows for the man to take control, and that mindset can build some major trust, and that's something that many women like about this.

The trust that's built here is something deeper than what many are used to. It's a form of trust that's quite explicit, and something that can be a bit jarring at first, but it's also something that can make a relationship better than before.

For women, the idea of taking control affects them in a different manner. Typically, it's normally seen that the man is the dominant one, and the female is the "feminine, submissive one." But that doesn't always have to be the case. If a woman takes control, it can give the woman a lot of confidence, and it gives them a sense of agency. Plus, let's be real, men find it really sexy when women are in control.

For many men, the idea of being "on top" psychologically all the time is exhausting. Following those roles constantly can be quite hard. Maybe a woman wants to take control, or the man likes it when the woman is on top. If that's the case, BDSM is perfect, because the roles themselves have no gender, which makes it even more awesome!

With BDSM, it often means that the dynamic changes with many couples too. They don't feel like they have to follow some sort of "mold" and instead, they can experiment. Many people don't like this because they've got the ingrained mindset that women are supposed to be submissive, and men dominant. But, learning to play with these roles, and even switching them up, can give them a lot of confidence. It's quite fun.

With BDSM, you need to have an open mind. That's the biggest part of it, and you've got to have an open mind when it comes to sexuality. You should make sure that anything you do try is something that won't harm yourself or your partner. In fact, If you do harm it's something illegal. However, consensual pleasure involving this type of play can make a huge difference in a relationship, and it can start to change the way people feel, and it can affect your relationship dynamic in various different ways.

For many women, this does give them that sort of control and confidence that they want to have, and it can have sex even more amazing for both the man and the woman. So, BDSM is something that can help, and it's not something "dirty" or "taboo" but instead something extremely fun.

Why This Play is Good

This play can change the mental state of your body, in different types of ways.

That's because, when you're doing this, you're actually releasing endorphins in the body. Every time you're in pain, or there is some type of experience is occurring, your body will release these "happy hormones" and you'll feel really good.

This can be extremely liberating for both the dom, and the sub, since it can release these feelings in both of their minds.

Now, when you're doing this, you should always make sure that you both are cool with exploring them. But, when you do relinquish this type of control, allow for your partner to do the bidding, this creates trust.

Trust is something that many people struggle with sometimes. They feel like they always have to be on guard, or in control. But sometimes not being in control is pretty great. Allowing another person to consensually and safely take control can be an amazing feeling. There isn't anything "wrong" with that. Being pampered and taken care of in different ways, allowing your body to feel different sensations, and overall pleasure in this form can be quite liberating, and extremely stimulating.

If you've never done this before, it's always worth a try. It can be quite different, but it is pretty nice.

This chapter discussed what BDSM is, and why people engage in it. It's quite liberating, and stimulating, and you'll be able to really get a feel for this whenever you get started in this activity.

Chapter 2: Important things to Remember when it comes to BDSM

There are some important things that you must do when it comes to BDSM. These various elements are integral to a pleasurable experience, and all too often, people forget about this. You need to make sure that when you're putting this together, it is perfect for each of you, so that everyone has what they want.

If you're doing this with someone who isn't a serious partner but instead you're looking for a dom, you will put together a "contract." In essence, this is everything that you agree to, and if you violate this contract, you can terminate the relationship. It's sort of like a business agreement.

Remember when Christian Grey demanded Anna to follow the contract? Yeah, you don't demand these things. You don't do what he did, but instead, we are going to start with everything that you need to know before you begin with this, and different elements that will make a huge difference in the success of this relationship.

You're both on Equal Ground

The biggest thing that you must remember when you're doing this, is that you're both on equal ground when it comes to this, and the distribution of power. When you're doing this with your domestic partner, you also want to be on equal ground, but if you're searching out a dom, or wanting to try this, you should keep this in mind.

In essence, this means that the power is equal between you both when you're discussing various things.

Now, this doesn't mean that in the scene you have equal power. That would mean that you aren't really experiencing BDDM. BDSM involves relinquishing some control in the form of a dom and a sub, but when you're negotiating, you always, ALWAYS, need to make sure that you're both on equal playing feelings.

This is important because it will address the wants and the needs that not only you have, but what the other persons wants and needs as well. This is very important for both parties, because if you're both not on equal footing, this is how upsets and problems happen.

When you're negotiating this type of contract in the submissive role, you might run the risk of relinquishing your own personal power, and consenting to things that you normally wouldn't consent to.

But, if you're doing this with a partner, you both sit down and talk it out. Discuss what you want and need, discuss the aftercare procedures, and discuss anything that you feel is important to your personal needs. This goes for doms, subs, and switches too. Seriously, talk this out before you get yourself into a situation you don't want to be in.

Opt in

When you're putting together a BDSM relationship, whether it be both you and your partner, or an actual contract, opting in is a very important thing. In essence, when you "opt in" to something, it's what you're saying yes to.

In essence, it's what you want, and what you don't want when you're putting together a BDSM contract, you always want to add in the opt in parts that you're into, rather than just the opt out method.

Lots of times, we only focus on the opt out parts of relationships, which are essentially the off limits part of this, and the deal breaker. If you do this, you'll say no to things you don't want, but you might also not say what you do want, and that can then make things a little more blurry.

When you're only thinking of what you don't want to do, it can make the whole relationship a lot more confusing, and create way more misunderstandings.

Instead of focusing what you don't want, focus on what you want, and also stipulate anything that you're consenting to, and only talk about what you consent to. If it's not in agreement, then you know what you do? You don't do it. You know exactly what you're getting into, and what you've consented to, and you'll only do what you've consented to, nothing more nothing less. That will give you safety with your partner, and you'll want to create that safe atmosphere for best results.

With this, you should ways make sure you talk about what you do want. Maybe you've had a fantasy. Talk to your partner, communicate it, and don't just talk about everything that you won't do, but instead opt in and talk about what you will do.

Consent is Sexy!

One of the biggest things that you should make sure that you have with any BDSM situation, is consent.

Why is consent so important? Because if you don't have it, it can spell bad news for you. For example, lots of times people don't realize that consent, when not given, can lead to some very bad repercussions, including rape accusations, and it can teeter on the edge of abuse.

This is why the BDSM community tends to get a bad name. People think that it is abuse, or something like that. But, with any BDSM situation, scene, or the like, you always need consent.

You want to make sure you have consent when it comes to each of these situations, whether it be from the person themselves during this, or even just in writing before the scene. This is why the contracts are important, because they will help you specify just what you need to know, and what's good, and what's not so good.

This goes with any sexual situation really. If you have consent, you should be fine. If you don't, then simply just don't do it. It's as simple as that, and you shouldn't make it more complicated than what it is. It's a simple yes or no answer, and if you have full-on consent, you'll feel better.

Get some specifics

Along the same lines as the previous section, you want to be specific. Lots of times, people think they are being specific enough, but that's not the case. Typically, when you're doing this, you should always be specific in what you like, and what you're writing down. You should watch out for vagueness, since that is a major problem with many contracts that people begin with.

You want to make sure that you're VERY specific when it comes to this. You should always teeter on the edge of more specific than vague. You should make sure that everything, from the rules, to the acts, are various elements that you do consent to. You should always give great detail to the acts that you're cool with, so that you don't misunderstand period, and both you, and the partner you're with, know what they want, and what is allowed in the BDSM relationship, and what isn't cool.

This even goes with what you're interested in when it comes to how you do certain things. For example, let's take that you want to be spanked. Problem is, there are *a lot* of different ways to get spanked, whether it be with a flogger, paddle, hands, or even other instruments. You want to be very specific in how you want to be spanked, for example, maybe you are cool with hands, but not with a paddle, or maybe vice versa due to trauma, but you like the feeling of being spanked. You may also want to be retained. How clothed you are even comes into play when it comes to specifics. It's a bit surprising that even clothed and unclothed specifics are a part of this, but often, there are some BDSM acts that involve being completely clothed, and it creates a different sensation. Sex always isn't an element either, so it can be a factor as well. Just be as specific as possible, and you won't have a problem.

Know the hard limits

Let's take a moment to discuss hard limits. These should always be considered before you get into this type of lifestyle.

Hard limits are essentially sexual acts that are not to be done. Period. No matter what, you never do these with your partner. The thing about these, is just like fetishes and kinks, everyone has different ones. For example, some don't like peeing, some aren't into bondage, and some may not like knife play. All of these things are different acts, and if it's a hard limit, you don't do it, no matter what the circumstance. If you don't follow the words and do this, you're breaking a huge part of your contract, and you can terminate this agreement. Not to mention, it's really uncool if you don't give respect to a person's hard limits.

Hard limits should be discussed before any play begins. You don't leave this to be discussed during the act itself, but doing it beforehand will ensure that everyone is on the same page. You want to make sure this is all discussed, and everyone is happy.

RACK

One acronym that you may see when you're learning more about BDSM, is RACK. RACK doesn't refer to an actual rack, or a term for a woman's bosom, but it's actually a very important part of preparing for a scene. This means Risk Aware Consensual Kink, which in essence are the guidelines to make sure that people know of what they're consenting to in terms of danger. There is another, called SSC, which means you keep the activities sane, safe, and consensual. The purpose of this is to make sure everyone is fulfilled and happy, and only gives them pain when they want it, not actual harm that could hurt others.

Some don't like SSC because it leaves various elements much vaguer, and some argue that it's much more open to interpretation, since often, those that are considered "sane and safe" in the community might be different from society. However, RACK gives the acknowledgement that there are different things that people consider sane and safe in a sense, and it essentially allows those who indulge in this to know what risks these activities take. It gives people much more flexibility to the ones that engage in this. There are some who like to play when they're under the influence, which if it's consensual that can happen, but there is a significant level of risk to it.

Both of these terms essentially tell the same thing: do stuff with consent, and make sure both parties know what they're getting into, and take the precautions that they need to for the activity itself. The intent is there, the rest can be semantics that you can debate for a long time. However, you need to remember here that you should choose the definition that works best for you. You should choose the word that gives you the best comfort and experience.

Safe words

Let's talk about safe words! Safe words are words that both your partner and you agree upon before you begin any sort of BDSM act. This is a word that allows you to feel safe, and assured whenever you're beginning any sort of risk play. If you use this word, it's essentially a safety word, and it's a very important part of BDSM.

Why is it important? Well, if you're trying out something new, such as maybe you're getting into a new type of bondage, and you feel uncomfortable, or maybe it's a little too traumatic for some, you can say this word, and immediately the play partner will stop what they're doing. It basically puts a complete stop to the whole scene.

Now, you have the contract, right? All contracts can change if there is something that makes you immediately uncomfortable to the point where it doesn't make you feel good. This is good for when you're in a situation where you're unsure of if you are cool with this or not.

But, it's got another use. You can determine the safe word as a form of "safety call." This is something you should discuss with a trusted friend before you begin a BDSM act with someone. You can, if you feel like you're in a situation where it's unsafe or meeting a new play partner, implement this. The safety call is used as well if you meet a new play partner that you like. This is just a safety check so that you're not in a risky situation.

If everything is all good, arrange to call during a time, and say the coded word to your friend. This coded word will say in essence that you're safe and comfortable with the partner you're with, and they don't have to worry. You've consented to this new BDSM scene with this person.

Now, if they don't receive the call, they can call the police at this point, and if you're in a high-risk situation, this is encouraged. Now, don't be a bit spacy with these calls, since they can save your life, and if you are spacy and forget, it can cause a lot of awkwardness when you have the police banging down on your door during a safe and consensual act, and it can cause some controversy. It's something that you should use when meeting new partners.

Even so, safe words are very important, and you need these in order to have a great time with a new person.

The difference between BDSM and Abuse

When it comes to BDSM, it's very important to recognize whether you're engaging in BDSM, or if it's abuse. There is a very clear line, and a huge difference between both of these things, many don't actually know the difference between each of these.

However, if you know about the difference and have a more informed idea of it, you'll be able to have a better lifestyle for yourself, and for others. Remember, BDSM doesn't involve sex all the time, but if you're having sex, you should always use protection with this.

So, what's the big difference between them? Well, they are as follows:

- BDSM is sensations used for pleasure, whereas abuse is damage be mental, physical, or emotional to another person
- BDSM is consensual power exchange that brings empowerment to both parties, but abuse usurps one person's power
- BDSM creates excitement in the partner, but it causes most people to be afraid of the partner they have
- Before you do anything, BDSM must have agreements put in, but abuse is much vaguer, and many don't know how, when, or even what will happen, creating a mystery
- BDSM relies upon trust, but abuse destroys all of this
- BDSM is used to help fulfill the desires of both people within a safe space, but abuse is cruel and very violent
- BDSM relies on open communication and support for both people, so they can talk about the emotions and thoughts, but abuse doesn't have any support

You can see the differences here, and knowing the difference can make a huge change in the different aspects of BDSM when it comes to yourself, your partner, and the like.

There is also the aspect of people assuming BDSM are mentally ill. Some people may suffer from mental illness, but there are people in the community itself that do. It's something that doesn't occur only in certain circles, or because of the action, but family history, genetics, and the like are definitely the cause in cases. Many times, if you are suffering from mental illness, it's important to seek some help.

There is research that has shown that many people are against the idea of getting mental health assistance from services because of BDSM, but it's important that if you're suffering from this, you get the assistance that you need.

This goes for partners as well. Many people in the BDSM community don't have the support, and if you have a partner that's needing support, make sure they get the professional help that they desires, so that it can help with the comfort of the community, and help reduce the stigma of mental illness, along with bias against kinks and such. It's important to keep an open mind when engaging in BDSM, since it can be used to help others overcome trauma. Lots of times, people use this as a means to escape, and it can help with that, so definitely keep an open mind.

Moral conditions regarding BDSM

There are some moral conditions that you should always keep in mind when engaging in BDSM. Here are the important moral conditions that you should engage in:

- Always be ethical: don't just say this, but actually follow the ethics. If you're not ethic in your playtime, or in other areas of your life, it reflects on yourself, and the community, so always try to be ethical.

- Know what you're getting into: understand the kink you're doing, because you're accountable for any risks that happen, and make sure to practice the kink before using it on people.
- Create a safe environment: always minimize risks, and know the environmental dangers of different elements, including any equipment you use, any candles that are lit, and even electricity. Make sure when you're done, you sanitize and clean every equipment and toy you use. You should also know about the partners you're with, the fantasies, hard limits, and any physical and emotional limitations, and learn to respect this.
- It's not therapy: you're not a therapist, and neither is your partner, unless you have that as a part of it. If there are issues you need help with, get some actual help, not just BDSM.
- Be honest: you should always be open and honest with your partner. This is a trust thing, and make sure you don't leave out anything that's necessary, and never make promises you can't keep, or pretend you're someone else, outside of roleplay obviously.
- Never harm a person: there is a difference between delivering pain, and harming someone, so make sure you're conscious of what's going on, and stay within the boundaries. If you inflict any punishment that is unintentional, indiscriminate, or any unwanted harm to a person, that's a red flag, and makes you look like an abusive person, or a bully, and make sure that if pain is done, it's intentional and consensual.
- Respect the privacy of others: not everyone is able to be open about their lifestyle choices. Be aware of the situation and don't out it unless they want you to.

- Take care of yourself too: you matter! You should always take care of your own health, whether it be emotionally, physically, or mentally, before engaging in this. It's a stability thing, and you should make sure that you do this for yourself, and your partner.
- Make sure the experience is complete: don't begin unless you see to what they need, and provide what they need when they come back from the headspace that might happen. You want to see to any emotional and physical needs that are important here.

Knowing these ethics is important, so do this before you begin.

Finding a fetish partner

If you're interested in finding a fetish partner, and you've already assessed what you want, and the attributes, let's discuss where you should go to find one. There are a few options.

You can first go online to find this. Sites like Fetlife are good to help you understand the lifestyle more, and it allows you to find ones that have specific preferences, and it's more under the radar.

It's got its advantages and disadvantages, where you can talk to a lot of kinky people around different areas, and you can connect with them, flirt with them, or even try to connect. This can also be done anonymously.

However, there is the anonymity of it, and some people are less accountable for what they do, and they might try to spread gossip. Plus, sometimes it's safer to meet these people online in an open place before anything else.

There are a lot of BDSM sites out there, so it's a good option.

Munches are another option. You might wonder what they are, but in essence they're a get together of people who are kinky to discuss interests and ideas, and it's usually done in a casual place. Most of the times these happen once or twice a month. Social networking sites and kink stores will tell you, and this is a great way to meet kinksters.

You can also use Findamunch.com, which tells you of munches all over the place, and if you know of a munch that's happening that you can't find online, you can put it on the site, and connect with others.

Finally, there are educational groups and events that talk about teaching aspects of BDSM, and this is a great way to meet different kinksters and expand what you know. This is also a good time to mingle, but don't expect these to have sex there, and typically it's a respectful atmosphere.

When it comes to BDSM, understanding the different aspects of it is quite important, and being able to create an atmosphere that's good for yourself and for others, is quite nice, and it makes a huge difference.

Sometimes, understanding how to be a good dom can be hard. If you're someone that hasn't engaged in BDSM before, you may wonder how to be a good one, to make it desirable for a partner, and you want to make sure that you do this right.

Everyone has their own desires, and sometimes, having the ability to push these is what makes a huge difference. Before you begin, sometimes accepting your kinks, and developing maturity with it is a good start, and if you're not able to talk about this, then you can't explore them safely. You should learn how to explore this in a safe manner, and also the different ways to be a good dom for another person. Often, when you're being a dom, you want to make sure that you do this right. As a dom, you'll be in control of whatever scene you're in, making the choices for the sub, and you're going to make sure results are gotten.

Many think being a dom is just being in control, just telling others what to do. That's NOT what it is, and there is a lot more responsibility and work to it, so you're able to create the results you want. This chapter will go over why people submit, and various factors to keep in mind when you're a dom.

Why Submit?

You may wonder why, as a dom, anyone would want to submit. After all, lots of times it involves offensive, degradation, and humiliation. Many times, people might think that it's a bit hard to be this way as a dom. However, it's more of a respect thing, and if you do this right, you'll definitely create a great relationship.

The concept that comes from this is based on a desire to be healthy, positive, and good to your person. Often, the pain and degradation are used on the sub with their consent. They want this. **You're doing this, but you're doing it in a respectful way.**

Yes, you may say those words, **but** you're never hurting the sub. You love them to some degree, and there isn't **any anger, disgust, or hate behind your words.**

The reason why people submit, is because they trust you as a dom, and you're in essence taking responsibility for the sexual scene. It's up to you for the other to have a good time, and you get pleasure out of making sure the other has a good time. If you're good, you'll take the burden off the other, so they can experience. They can shut off their mind, and submit.

Submitting is actually a way of letting go to become free. This trust isn't something that's lightly, and if you're scared of doing this, you should consider the type of limits you have as a partner.

With this, you're in control, and you make the choices, give punishments, and give praise when it's appropriate. The paradox is that the sub is in power. The sub chooses what they want and don't want, and they have the final say. The only choice a sub makes in this is to choose to give the power to another. You always want to make sure that it's willfully given.

You're not in Charge

One thing that you should realize, and one thing you'll have to accept, is that you may be "in charge" but you also are not the one with the final say on what gets to be done and not done. You're kind of like a co-author in essence to the scene, or a story. You're with the person writing it, but you're not the full-on author. The author is the sub, since they are the ones that have the final say on what they like, don't like, and they are in charge of what you do in a sense. They submit power, but again this power paradox comes in where they're in charge.

It can happen where you do power trip, and this can create an altered state, which is called a dom space or a top space. The power dynamic is here though. As a dom, you get sensual sensation and experience from being in charge. You like being in charge. But, you are following what the sub wishes, and it fits into your own personal desires. You're not just dominant because the other is calling you master. You may not even look like the dom in terms of traditional elements. It's based solely on listening, taking action, and stepping back. You're in control of the scene, and of yourself, and the partner is the one that's trusting you, so remember that.

Communication is important

Second rule always have open communication. If you want to be considered a good dom, and not someone that the sub looks at with a bit of a disgusted look after the scene is over, and judging whether or not that was abuse, you have to make sure you are communicative.

This includes before, during, and after. Before is the contract, and you follow the sub's wishes. You derive pleasure from being on top, and making your partner feel good.

During the scene, you listen to how the partner is. If they're good, then keep going. If it looks like you should change it, then do so. If you hear the safe word, you stop the scene period. If the scene is completed, you give aftercare to the sub as needed, communicating what could be better, and what the sub liked and didn't like.

If you're a good dom and engages in communication, your sub will be quite happy, and you'll do a great job.

Be safe!

Always be safe when it comes to these. This is obvious, but remember that the submissive partner is completely trusting you, and their physical safety is a big part of it. You may feel a bit of worry about whether or not the partner is fine, so make sure that it's safe for them.

This goes for many different things. You should discuss what contraception and safe sex the sub wants, any tools used and making sure you know how to use them to make the scene as safe as they can. While both need to make sure everything is done with a proper manner, the dominant needs to check in with the scene, listen to the safe words and any other communication that should be there. You should make sure that safety is implemented even when a person is gagged, or they can't speak. Because once it begins, emotions happen, endorphins start to come about, the roles can lose the person, and if both parties forget, this can cause a huge issue later on remember that as a dom, you're responsible for the reactions.

If you're doing any bondage play, always have safety scissors to get the person out of this. Make sure you practice RACK, preventing any other sexual risks that can happen, and the like. Words and a conversation should be had beforehand so that you're all safe, and you have a great experience.

Don't make mistakes

While some believe mistakes can always happen, when it comes to being a dom, it's almost unacceptable. It might seem like a contradiction, but sometimes, if you make sure you have the safety precautions in, you'll be able to accomplish what you want, with precision.

You should, as a dom make sure to push the limits, without breaking them or going too far with this. You should push this as hard as possible, and then getting the sub to come begging for more. If they don't come back, you did it wrong.

You should remember that it can be dangerous, and just because you see a porn video that is hot, doesn't mean you should try this during a scene. If it's discussed beforehand, you should be fine, but always make sure you know the person's limits, and cater to them.

Be honest

This is another huge part. Honesty is important, not just in big lies, but in this type of lifestyle, it's everything.

There are two ways you're honest, and they are:

- Honesty with yourself
- Honesty with the sub

You should know exactly what you want, need, and what you should avoid. When it comes to your subs, you should make sure relay what you want and need, and you should make sure that you give them what they want in return. You shouldn't lie about this, telling them what you think they should hear. They want the truth, no matter how hard it is always be honest with this, because it could bite you in the ass in the future.

Honesty also goes for the sub as well. It's not just the sub telling you something and then going on with what they're doing. You want to make sure they're telling the truth, and you want to make sure that you're accurately and correctly breaking the limits of the sub. This is the only way to make sure that you get the correct information.

You should make sure that honesty is a big part. Some subs may not lie, but they might be ignorant of the limits. This isn't any sort of insult, but it's impossible to know how someone will react to a situation. They might not think they will react to something, but then they do. That's why safe words are used too.

If something does go wrong, you stop the scene when you hear the safe word, and you make sure that you're calm, healthy, and you're safe, and then if there is an upset, you discuss what happened, and if it was your fault, accept it, and you should make sure you give support and compassion to the other person. You shouldn't expect to continue the scene, especially if it did create an upset. If you do make a mistake, realize that if you screw up, you'll need to pay for it.

Various elements to remember:

There are a few elements to remember, and they are as follows:

- As a dom, you care for your sub and have the best interest at heart
- Remember, you're not a sadist and egomaniac. You're not ordering or hurting the sub, but instead pushing limits together
- You have to take responsibility, step up to the plate, and take control
- You should make sure not to confuse sadism and masochism with dominance and submission, they're different things
- The dominant is a leader, doer, and someone who provides for another

- A dominant needs to accept that submissive will be needy. If the dom isn't ready to take on emotional needs, then they won't do well with this
- You can't be selfish and be a dom. If you are cruel, it's essentially playing good with people
- The dom will control the different aspects of the scene, including orgasms, since it could be pleasure that is earned
- Some doms are sadists, but not all are. This is based on needs
- You may notice a submissive will try to fight back and rebel. This is testing dominant limits, and you want to keep control, not become emotional or anything, and be in charge
- When you do discipline and punish a sub, you should make sure that this is fair, without emotion, relevant, and controlled. You can reinforce the positions at this point, and it will give submissive that feeling of safety. The sub after should feel positive, and the dom should try to do what's best for the sub
- The relationship is balance. For every single painful action, it should be counterbalanced with a positive action. Don't let this go out of whack
- A good dom is working to make shy submissive grow and improve, and the dom won't use the power granted for just your own sexual gains, but instead create rules to help the sub get better direction, and enrich them

And that, is how to be a good dom. Follow this, and you'll be much happier as a result.

Chapter 4: How to be a Good Sub

We talked about how to be a **good dom**. There is a lot of responsibility there. But, did you know that you need to **know** how to be a good sub as well? Often, people don't know how to be a good **sub,** and this can be a bit of a problem, and often, lots of new subs may walk into **this** with the wrong idea.

The thing with BDSM, is that it's **quite** powerful, almost magical in a sense, and some people don't realize the **full** power of this until they're in it. You may find out that you don't like the **reaction** that can happen, when you thought it would be fine. There are a few things **that** you can learn to be a good sub without completely sacrificing your personality, or losing yourself in the process. Here they are, and various aspects **to keep in mind.**

Exercise your power within your role

When it comes to being a sub, **you may** believe that you just let the dom do whatever the hell they want **to you** here's the thing, it's more than just that. You may love being bent over and **spanked** to the point where you cum. But there is so much more to that. Lots of **times,** being a sub means that you're giving yourself up and handing over the safety **to another** person for some time. That's a great power, and it comes with a great **responsibility.**

You need to learn to play the **role of** a sub, and being strong with this. You first of all need to have good discretion **when** it comes to choosing the dom. You want to choose one that won't just **belittle** and undermine you, making you feel bad. When you choose a dom, you **want** someone who is worthwhile, who will protect you. You're in charge of your **own** health and wellbeing when you're getting into these situations.

While yes, the dom does ultimately have the responsibility *during* the scene, it's after and before that's on you. You want to make sure you won't be chided into things you don't want to do. You want to choose partners that will help them get better, via complimenting and allowing you as a sub to challenge your roles, allowing you to grow as a good sub in the BDSM experience.

It might seem weird that you can grow as a sub. Well guess what, you can grow as a person. You'll be able to choose a good person that's responsible for you, and someone that you can respect and aspire to be. You can let this person take control, but you'll also enjoy it, and you will want to choose someone that makes you feel safe and cared for.

Do communicate awareness

If you do have any problems when it comes to your physical and mental state, you need to communicate these to your dom. Communication is the key to success, yes, and if there are any vulnerabilities, triggers, or the like, you must communicate these to your dom.

For example, let's say you're about to form a contract with a dom. You don't like being choked, due to personal issues in the past. If that's the case, you should always communicate this to your dom. You should as well, if you're trying out a new kink, and you find out that it really doesn't sit well with you, you should exercise your judgment and tell your dom how you're feeling.

If needed, you should also utter the safe word if you don't want that boundary pushed anymore, if you want it to be stopped. That safe word is there for you, and you should always make sure that you use it. This is an example of how just in control you are.

You may think you have no control, but as said before in the previous chapter, you've got a hell of a lot more control than you imagine. You want to make sure you exercise it, and use it as needed if you feel unsafe.

Take care of your mental stability

Being a sub isn't just because you need someone to pick you up and take care of your mental stability. That's on you. You're not using your dom as a sort of prince charming to save you from yourself, because that's not the purpose of this. You shouldn't also have this because you want the dom to save who they are through you.

If you think about it, that's how 50 Shades was, and that's not BDSM. That's not how this works. BDSM is supposed to be for both of you, and it's an experience that should create comfort, fun, and amazing orgasms. If you have reservations and any mental afflictions that you feel need to be worked on before you get into it, then it's on you to ensure that you take care of yourself.

Sometimes some subs end up giving up their personality, and it's what they seek in this type of relationship. But, if you're not comfortable with that, you need to continue to make sure that you're being yourself, even when you're submissive.

This is also on you, knowing what you want to alter, what you want to share with the person you're with. Partners will ask questions, and you should be ready to give answers to this that are honest, and if you want this to actually work out. If you're weak, evasive, and not at the forefront when discussing this with them, that's how problems are created. Being open now will save your bacon later on, so make sure that you do this.

Remind yourself that this IS risky

Sometimes, you may think that there isn't that much risk to what you're doing, even something as small as bondage. But, it does matter a lot when you're looking to be interested in what you're exploring. Things that are simple are risky, even if you think they're fine.

Let's take bondage. If you're using something small, even so much as a scarf or tie, this still poses some risks. You can get minor injuries from bondage, including chafing, maybe even a little bit of broken skin, and even circulation issues.

There are some instances where if you don't know this, it can even leave you dead. If you bind someone in the correct manner, you'll reduce the risk of this. There is a right way and a wrong way to tie up someone, and if you aren't prepared for the unexpected, such as maybe having a pair of safety scissors nearby, the unexpected does happen, and they find out the hard way.

As a sub, you need to make sure that you're educated, and your dom is educated, and you want to make sure that you do have a good education on what is going on. If they're not educated, that puts you in risky situations. If your dom doesn't know how to do something, that puts you at risk, so you should make sure you educate, not just by reading, but by talking, asking questions, and getting answers as to how to do various things. That way, you'll be able to recognize when something is wrong.

The more inexperienced you are, the less prepared you are to deal with the unexpected. If you don't want to call your best friend in a panic because you're in the emergency room due to a mistake made in a session, you should definitely make sure that you do educate yourself. Learn from this, and understand that

BDSM is quite powerful, and a reaction might come about that you're not ready for.

Often, the reason why this happens is because we are exploring repressed desires, and as a sub, you run into something called a "sub frenzy" which is in essence like a kid in the candy store, demanding you get everything now. You must protect yourself from yourself when you get like this. That's why, always educate, and if you're doing something new with some risk, you always ALWAYS make sure that you get a dom that does have an idea on how to do something. The last thing you want, is an accident.

Watch out for certain Doms

Just like with any person out there, there are types of doms you get the hell away from, and we will go over a couple of the types to avoid.

Your two top types to get away from are the following:

- The creepy dom
- The fresh meat dom
- The collective dom

Now, creepy dom is obvious as to why you stay the hell away from them. Don't want a creep? Don't find this dom.

The fresh meat dom is also someone that you should avoid too. This is someone that gets turned on by someone who is new, and they are *persistent* about following you for different reasons.

Lots of times, these ones are super inexperienced as well, to the point of dangerous in the community. They will talk the talk and they'll try to win you over because you aren't experienced either. They will do everything possible to get you, even to the point of hiding the truth.

Now, there are newbie doms, just as there are newbie subs. But, the difference is that these people will misrepresent themselves, and they won't try to actively improve the knowledge, and understand the different aspects of BDSM. They refuse to learn, and instead talk big freaking game and they can hurt a lot of partners. They may even hurt you if you choose to take this risk.

This also will violate the safe, sane, and consensual elements that are put there in BDSM. It's not something you want, and you should get the hell out of there. This guy could be a wannabe, maybe not even a dom but is using this to get laid. He probably thinks that subs are easy, and they will do a lot of kinky things that older girlfriends won't do. They'll try to pressure you into trying things that you're not comfortable with.

They also may think, if it's a dominant dude, that unlimited blowjobs are on demand. Which is definitely not the case. You should get the hell away from this kind, because they're not interested in meeting your personal needs whatsoever.

Now, there is another type of dom that you may want to avoid as a personal measure. This is the experienced dom that likes to find fresh meat, mostly because it's a rush. You're inexperienced, and he likes that. he likes to introduce newbies to new sensations, and he likes the initial delight of helping you through these new sensations and passions, which is quite nice. In essence, this is a dom that gives you fun, experience, and a lot of excitement, but that's just it. This is a temporary thing, which is what you'll need to learn. They are amazing teachers, so if you want to learn, go here, but the truth is, lots of times these domes do pose a risk to your heart, since they already have a steady submissive and don't want to trade. If you seek this out immediately, you're going to hit the harsh reality that you'll have an amazing experience, but no connection. You may think this dom is your soul mate, but the reality is, chances are they probably aren't, and it's going to be quite a problem for you when that its.

The Catch-22 of all of this, is that a sub wants to find that person that they can go gaga for. Subs tend to fall into the tendency of this, since the appetite is enormous for a dom. The more a sub submits, the more control they give up. This may cause a sub to fall in "love" with their dom in a sense. It's part of the control aspect.

This actually does go into the part stated before about preserving your mental state. This includes, not falling in love with the first dom you have, unless you two have a super killer connection, and they're the one. If they are, then ignore this and be on your merry way.

A good dom can change your life interactions. You may feel like they're the one. Again, feeling like they're the love of your life, the dom "soulmate" in a sense. However, you'll find out a little ways down the road that it isn't the case. The initial encounters with the dom kind of might feel like the "honeymoon" experience with them. You'll have amazing connection, passion, and excitement that comes at the beginning of the relationship. Typically, the experienced dom knows of this, and they've dealt with this before. This can cause a lot of pain for a sub when it ends. It can hit you very hard, which is why you need to preserve your own mental state. Don't give everything up for an experienced dom that you don't have a connection with besides a lustful one. It can be hard to discern the difference between being in love with someone, and being just a mere plaything. It can be a very painful period of disillusionment for someone, and for you. If you don't understand d the dynamics, understanding that there is a difference between mere play and a connection, you're going to hit the ground fast, and hard.

This is something that, as a sub you need to watch out for.

Finally, and on a lighter note, you want to avoid the collector dominant. This is someone that, as a newbie sub, you should learn to avoid. They already have a ton of submissives, and you're just another part of the harem. If you go into this with open eyes, and no connections or strings attached, that's fine, but you should keep your hands on your heart and keep the heart out of this. That's because the sub can find themselves in a relationship that's entangled, and it may involve a lot of sacrifices at the end of the day.

This is mainly what to avoid as a newbie sub. You should always make sure you find one that you're comfortable with, and understand what you're there for.

Tips to being a better submissive

There are a lot of ways to improve being a better submissive. A sub should remember that they want to make the dom's life easier, but not harder for people. Often, thinking about what the dom needs all the time, and fulfilling it, will give them great pleasure. Obviously, sexuality and submission based on the contract is the obvious one, and there are probably different rules that you've implemented as well. That can create a good relationship with the dom, but there are some other things that can help you be a good submissive, and allow you to really get the most out of it.

These are things normally that you should do, but it's a good way to please your dom, and can make you feel good.

- Get some good sleep
- Exercise in a regular manner
- Eat well and preserve a healthy diet
- Dress in a proper way, possibly in line with the contract, such as a collar
- Having good grooming and hygiene

These are all obvious things in a sense, but it does help you hold yourself to a better, higher standard of life.

You should definitely make sure that you strive to please the dom, but also have your own needs met as well.

Learn your Dom

You should definitely learn who your dom is, and also cater to their desires. It isn't an "obligation" or any contractual thing, but it's something that you, as a submissive, should be keen on doing. It's totally okay to learn how to please your dom.

You should learn the likes and dislikes, and the submissive should ask whenever they don't know on something. It's good to study your dom to know what they like and don't like. Sometimes journaling this is great.

If you know something that pleases the dominant, you should practice it, get better, and do it to please the dominant, because you'll feel better, and it does give a sense of thrill to please the dominant.

However, you should go deeper, learning about the dominant as a person. You should learn what they like, don't like, what makes them feel better, their favorite things. It does help you give a more intimate knowledge of the dom, and how to please them.

Dominants aren't always 24/7 sex. That's something that you may think when you initially get into this, but that's actually something that isn't the case. They like to see that you care about them, and it's something that you should also remember.

Get people to admire you

Being a submissive doesn't mean you should only be pleasing your dom, what you should also be doing is building good character. Dominants like when people admire the submissives, even if the people don't know. You should be honest and respectful, compassionate when needed, and also try to be understanding. These are basic human virtues, but here's the thing, when this gets back to the dominant, they'll be pleased, and this will make them happy.

You should go into life knowing that what you do, say, how you look and dress, and how you handle things does get back to the dominant, and it's a reflection of them. This can be quite difficult, but if you're generally a good person, this is quite nice. It's definitely something that you should also remember, because it'll reflect on you as well. If you look good, you'll feel good.

This chapter discussed how to be a better sub. It can be quite hard, but if you know how to do it, it'll make you feel better about doing this.

Let's take a moment to talk about all of the wonderful different BDSM examples, how to do them, and how you can do some of these actions. The range of these is from pretty light, to something that's much harder, so make sure that if you do this, discuss it with your dom or sub, and make sure they're cool with this, and it's not a hard limit.

Bondage

First, we have bondage, something that is pretty familiar with anyone. This can be done by the most beginner, or advanced of doms and subs. In essence, this is retraining your partner using anything from scarves, belts, ropes, Velcro, handcuffs, or even specialty hooks and clasps if you want to get fancy. Some like to be restrained, and if you want this, you should discuss it.

CBT

This is cock and ball torture. This is exactly what it sounds like. This is something that some male submissives like, and some female or male dominants like as well. In essence, the dominant will either bind, whip, or use something that has some force to it to step on the cock, and to torture them. This can even be done in heels if that's what the submissive wants.

Edgeplay

This is the riskier activities that BDSM does have. You may not be into this, but it can involve various activities, including knife play, breath play, and blood play. Usually, for something to involve edgeplay, it has to be something that could potentially harm another person.

You may not want to do this if it's not your cup of tea. It is very risky, since it does involve getting hurt, and blood and other fluids might end up causing issues, especially if you haven't been tested for STIs yet. You should be careful with this type of play, and only do this with someone who knows what the heck they're doing.

Fisting

This is something that's also not for the beginner, but might be a term that you've heard. In essence, it's when you stick an entire fist in your butthole or vagina. It feels good surprisingly, and it won't ruin anything, but it's something that more vanilla people might not be interested in. But, if you do this, make sure you use lube.

Impact play

Impact lay is something that involves any sort of hit, or impact against the body. This isn't just the backside, but also other parts of the body as well. Typically, with impact play, you think of spanking when you hear about it. But, it can also be using a cane, flogging, or even just slapping, and it can be other types of impacts as well. Some like to use objects normally not used as something in impact play.

Knife Play

This is another form of edgeplay, and in essence, it's knife sex. This is something that can be dangerous, and it's best to do it with someone that does respect your boundaries, and someone that you can trust. Lots of times, it doesn't even draw blood, but there is a psychological thrill, since the knife that's being passed over the body creates an adrenaline rush.

Needle Play

Now, this is another type of edgeplay, and it does involve possible blood because you're using needles on someone. Always make sure that they're sterile, and of a surgical grade. Also, do this with someone that knows what they're doing, and if you're having trouble finding someone, look into a professional dom for this, because you have to play it safe. It can involve putting this in an erogenous zone. If you've been curious, seek a professional for this.

Orgasm Denial

Not into needles or anything too crazy? Well, how about orgasm denial. In essence, this is the next level of sexual anticipation for those that are just dying to get off and they've had it forever. Lots of times, it involves having to deal with this the brink of orgasm, and then, you're stopped. This can be the best, but also the most frustrating thing, but it's a fun type of BDSM to try.

To do this is easy, and even if you're not getting into the harder kinks, you can do this. You can even try it with a partner. Get them to the edge, and then, right before they orgasm, you just stop, and then try once again.

Queening

Do you want your sub to treat you like a queen? This is the chance to do it! this is for women most of the time, since it's a term when a woman, such as the queen that the sub worships, sits on the sub's face. It's a pretty name for face sitting, which is often a huge part of dom and sub play. The queen might sit there for hours on end, and it's something that some people just really like.

Topping from the bottom

If you are a bratty sub, or maybe you like to top from the bottom, this is a fun one. It is when a bottom tries to take control of the scene, even though they should submit due to negotiations. For example, sometimes the bratty sub might try to fight the dom. It can be a bit of an annoyance, and it might create upset if not already discussed beforehand, but in ageplay scenes, such as daddy dom, little girl, you may see this a lot, where the sub may be bratty.

Waardenburg wheel

This is a metal pinwheel that you can try if you're getting ideas of stimulation for the sub. It's a little metal pinwheel that does look a bit scary, but that, combined with bondage and maybe some blindfolding, can create a great stimulation. You can use it on the erogenous zones of the body, including the nipples, but it's actually very interesting.

Some people do like it, and it is a medical device that's used originally to test out the different nerve reactions, but it's also used in BDSM.

It is used in something called medical play or doctor fetish, which we will describe here as well.

Medical play

As stated before, you can use medical instruments in the bedroom for medical play. These are scenes that often involve medical equipment, medical anesthetic, and even medial tools. Some people do find it arousing to be stimulated in this fashion, and with a doctor roleplay attached to it, it can be quite stimulating.

This can be a form of edgeplay as well, since it does involve both needle play and play piercing. So, if you do this, do be careful

Ageplay

You may have heard of daddy dom, little girl, or something along these lines. This is a form of play that involves a replay aspect that is vast in terms of ages. Lots of times, the dom is a caretaker for the person, and the sub is usually roleplaying a younger age. This can incest play, diaper play, and other types of various aspects. Obviously, everyone who engages in this is of age, but it's roleplay, and it's something that may be interesting.

Choking

For some, they get off to being choked. There are various risks associated with this, so you should always make sure that you know them before you begin.

There are some different types. There is blood choking, which is a much stronger version of this, where you choke someone to the point of passing out, and it restricts the blood flow to the brain. This is considered in many cases edgeplay, and often, it's something that may not be used quite a lot in the kink community.

On a much lighter scale is breath play. This is restricting breath, whether it be for a few seconds, or longer. There are risks involved with this, and it can be considered very dangerous, so only do this with a trusted dom, since it is technically edgeplay.

There is even some forms of choking and breath play that doesn't necessarily involve choking directly, but instead limiting the breath. For example, you have corsetry, or tight lacing. This explores an interesting exchange of power and fetish through changing the shape of a body with a corset, sometimes limiting the breath of the person who is being put into it.

Cupping

This is also called fire cupping in some circles, where you take some glass cups, and you put them across the skin. They're usually warmed, and they're made of glass. When they cool down, you pull them off, and it creates a vacuum, along with some hicky bruising that goes across the skin. If you do this hard, it also does have a tendency to break the skin as well.

Caning

Caning is a BDSM activity where you use a cane to strike a person. Often, this is on the broad and fleshy areas of the body, such as the butt, the back of the thighs and other places. Some like to have it across the bottoms of the feet as well.

Collaring

Collaring is when you have a collar around your neck, usually representing the identity of a submissive, or in a sense "owned" by the dom. It can be whatever meaning you want with this, or no meaning at all, but it does have some symbolism in BDSM. You may even see a collaring ceremony that goes on in the kink community, since it can showcase a serious commitment. In some cases, this can mean anything from a mere commitment with a dom, to even a seriousness to it that is on par with marriage and engagement. Some like to wear them during playtime, and it's something that some enjoy.

Understanding some of the different types of kinks and kinky play that can happen can help you determine what you want. Obviously, these are all varied in nature, and you don't have to do them, they're just some interesting types of play, and if you have an open mind, it can be quite interesting to learn about.

Bondage is probably one of the most popular forms of BDSM. However, lots of times it isn't just for sexual pleasure. There are different types of bondage to try, and we'll go over what those are, and even how to do it, along with some tips to make it awesome for you, and your partner.

Japanese Bondage

While you may be familiar with bondage in terms of holding another person in an enclosure or strapped to something, there is also Japanese bondage as well. This is a very popular type of bondage where you have the partner tied up in a very intricate and amazing pattern, all through the use of rope. Lots of times, this is more of an artistic means of holding a person in a bound, and it's actually an art form rather than just restraint. It's quite pretty.

It takes a little bit of time to learn it, but it's something you can learn and master in no time.

Leather Bondage

One thing you've probably seen when looking at bondage is well, leather. Leather, whether it be in the clothing, or even in the restraints, is something that many people like in terms of restraints.

They're much stronger than say silk, and they don't leave marks like rope does. It's a popular form of restraint that many like to use, and that, combined with other forms of leather items such as clothing and paddles, does make for a great addition to any scene. If you are someone who is a bit conscious of the animals, you can always get the vegan friendly options, or a faux leather to make up for this.

Mummification

Mummification is wrapping or, creating a mummy sort of part on the body, and it's a form of confining movement, and even limiting the sensory experience with this. You can use plastic wrap, rubber, fabric, or even saran wrap. This can create an interesting simulation, but always make sure you leave an area open for the person to breathe.

Why bondage?

Why is bondage so attractive to people? Well, people like it for various different types of reasons. For starters, being bound allows for some people to relax and calm down. It helps to reduce the insecurity and the worry that might be there typically, and it allows the person to have some pleasure without having to worry about giving back.

Some like the idea of struggle too, because it gives you some adrenaline, and it can be a bit thrilling.

Some also like the idea of blindfolding with bondage, because it will heighten your other sensations, and it does give a thrill of power. The person who ties the other up does have the feelings of power as well, and it can be quite attractive.

You may be curious about what to try initially. Well, there are some various means to do so, and we'll discuss for first-timers what you should do.

Remember, some people think that bondage is all about whips and chains, but that's not the case. It's something that does exist there, but you don't have to do that. Beginner bondage is something that you do on your own terms, and you should try it, see if you like it, and if you don't, then that's fine.

First Time ideas

When trying it for the first time, here are a few fun ideas to try out. It can be a bit scary, but they definitely can create a thrill that you'll enjoy:

- Tying yourself and your partner up with silk scarves and using teasing
- Tie up the up with something they can easily break off, and let them stay in the position
- Blindfolding during either sex, a massage, or even kissing
- Using fuzzy handcuffs, since they are padded to prevent chafing, and they don't close very far
- Getting those safety handcuffs that have the latch you can press
- Take it a little further by using hot and cold items that you can use to stimulate. Ice cubes, or even warm honey can be used, and you can try these by stimulating your partner with them while they're bound, or even blindfolded. It can be quite fun

When it comes to bondage, these are great to try out. You can always get better restraints and such overtime, but definitely make sure that you're able to do what you feel is comfortable for yourself and your partner.

Going from one level to the next

If you're still not comfortable with even that, you should first try out an even more basic form.

You can have the dominant one hold the partner's hand, pinning them across the mattress. You can feel if that's comfy, and if it is, you should definitely try maybe handcuffs the next time. You can try different ways to explore this, and be open about the positions. You should see what you like in a psychological sense when it comes to this type of erotic play.

When you begin with tying up the partner, you may first try to go with something like a shirt tie, or even a stocking. While they're good for blindfolding, they aren't ideal for tying a person up, because it might be a struggle to get off since they can't undo the knot in the tie. With tights, they're stretchy and nylon, which means that they get tighter while tied, and you can create a disaster.

One thing that you can use to make sure that nobody is freaking out when being tied up, is Velcro. Velcro, can be snapped, twisted, pulled in different ways, and it won't come free, but, you can literally snap it and pull the partner out of it if there is a problem. This also does work for anything with an easy release clip. It's something that's there to help the person undo this when the heat of the moment is there. While you may never even use it, sometimes it's better to have this, than nothing at all.

Safety Instructions

When you're tying someone up, you should definitely watch for a few cautions. Here they are:

- Don't do this with someone that's new, or you just met. You don't know if you can trust them, or if they're right, until you know them better, even if they are charming. So, don't use this on Tinder dates

- You shouldn't let the partner bully or coerce you into sexual practice that you're not into. Remember you always say no
- You should talk about this beforehand and have a plan. Talk about what you do and don't do. This should already be discussed if you have a contract
- Make sure that the safe word is there. If this is uttered, the dominant should get the submissive out of this, releasing them from the restraints
- Never tie anything around the neck, except for a collar, since this risks tissue damage, strangulation, or choking
- You should watch for gags as well. Make sure that the person has a breathable one, since these can be dangerous
- When you tie a person up, never leave them alone, and make sure they are comfortable, can breathe properly, and there isn't anything cutting off the circulation
- When making sure something is restrained, it's good to make sure you can fit two fingers into there. That way, circulation isn't cut off
- Don't try bondage in a remote location, since this could create an accident that leaves the one active injured, and the passive is tied up without getting help
- If you've never done this before, don't go to the complicated equipment. You should only use those if you're an expert, since they involve a lot of other safety issues as well.
- Always make sure that you engage in safer sex. You should use condoms if penetrating, and don't drink or do drugs when having sex, because this can

create serious health risks. You should **avoid** intoxication whenever possible.

This chapter discussed bondage, why you **may like** it, and some of the different types. It's best to learn from the bottom and start up, making sure that you have created the best atmosphere for your **partner**.

Chapter 7: Beginner BDSM Actions to Try

So, you've been reading a lot **about** some of the different elements of BDSM, and maybe you want to start playing **into** these fantasies. One of the biggest issues for many couples who begin with **this**, or even just on a singular basis with your own personal sexploration, is the **fact that** you probably think most of what's been discussed earlier is a little bit "much." While yes, you can work up to it, sometimes starting off slow, **and working** up to some of the heavier elements of play is important. If you've **been considering** light BDSM, then look no further. If you're a newbie, I highly suggest **choosing** one of these and incorporating it into your next play session, or even **when** having sex.

Lots of people paint BDSM as **stuff** you see in hardcore pornography, where the woman is doing something **very hard** on the body, such as maybe being bound in very tight restraints, and the guy is smacking her, maybe even punching her. But, that's very hard BDSM, and that **type** of play is often too much for many people. If you're a kinky person, or you've **wanted** to explore this, then try out these beginner BDSM tips to explore. **If** you find these too easy, then you can always look further into this.

Pulling hair

Hair pulling is a great way to get started with this. With hair pulling, you can be as hard, or as soft as you'd like. **You** should communicate, so that you don't go too heavy with this, but it's one of **the** best beginner BDSM actions to try, since you are in control. Do it maybe while you're being taken from behind, and see if that's what you enjoy.

Spanking (but light of course)

Now, with spanking, you've probably had a fantasy of this before. Maybe you've been patted on the butt in the past, but you want something a little bit more hardcore. That's totally an option, and one of the best things about BDSM, is the fact that with this action, you can start off soft, and then work your way up to it.

The best way to begin is always with your hands. The problem with paddles, floggers, and the like, is the fact that they tend to be a bit much for the average person to begin with, and you may end up accidentally hitting your behind a little bit harder than you expected with this. You should first use hands. If you feel like you want something more, move onto toys.

With spanking, the reason why people enjoy it, is both because of pain, and because of power. The pain starts to unleash endorphins into the body, making you feel good as well. Plus, having that position of power taken away from you and given to someone else is always a huge turn on for many women, so it's certainly something that many enjoy due to that.

Tying Up

Now, I don't suggest going out and getting industrial rope, or tying up your partner in some sort of intricate Japanese shibari, but what I do suggest, is using something soft that won't damage you.

Examples of that are scarves and ties, similar to what Christian Grey did, but obviously make sure you've got consent.

With handcuffs and rope, sometimes these can be tight, and it might end up chafing and hurting the skin. But, the cool thing about scarves, is that you have to really pull on this super tight in order to aggressively damage a person.

Now, if you do this, you should make sure that you can put two fingers into the area there so that you can avoid cutting off the circulation, which does do damage and can hurt the person, so definitely be mindful of this.

Aggressive Language

Now, if you're someone that wants to be called words in the bedroom, this is a great form of light BDSM.

However, I don't suggest being called names that can end up being a bit hurtful. Saying words such as slut, whore, wimp, brat, jerk, or even fuck if you don't use those words can be a good thing that you should try out.

However, it's also important to discuss what words are able to be used when engaging in aggressive language. Some girls like to be called filthy whores when engaging in BDSM, but maybe if you say that, the girl might get pissed off, and it can be a major turn-off and ruin the experience.

I do suggest before you begin, that you do discuss what words are good, and what words are bad. If some words make you feel bad, then you shouldn't use them. Remember, this is supposed to be pleasurable, so you want to make sure they're words that the other person wants to hear.

Restraints under the bed.

Okay, if you have ever wanted to try out restraints that you can use on the bed, get some of those under the bed restraints.

I do suggest that you make sure you at least have done scarves and moved up from this. For many people, this can be a bit harder than what they're used to, so you should take some time and figure out what the best level of restraint is. The under-the-bed restraints are often good because they give a bit of room and comfort, without possibly making it uncomfortable for the other person.

Incorporating Sir and Madam

Sometimes, even just saying this is something that is a nice beginner entry into BDSM. It often is good because it gives a bit of power to the other person, but it doesn't feel like you're totally relinquishing control to another. Plus, pet words that you use for the sub are good too, and are simple.

Biting

Biting is another great one if you're looking to begin with BDSM, but here's the thing, you need to discuss how hard you want to bite.

Some people are cool with marks, other people don't like them. If you're not someone that is cool with having a little souvenir left behind, that you may need to cover for your next business meeting, always talk to your partner and tell them no marks. You need to also talk about how hard you bite too, because some people bite pretty hard, and if you get chomped down too hard and don't like it, it can cause an upset between both of the partners.

Before you begin, make sure when you're going over what's cool, and what's not cool, you talk about this, so that you know where each of you stand before you begin. You always talk about stuff first before you do get into it, because there is nothing more freaking awkward than finding out someone hates the feeling of being bit down too hard, and then you end up upsetting them.

Sub and Top Role Play

This is mostly just looking to get more of the sub and dom dynamic together. This can involve begging, a little bit of restraint, or even trying to put the other person in a submissive position. If you have the girl on top, she's riding, and maybe she restrains your hands and then tells you to beg for movement, that's an example of this.

This is something that's super simple, and it can be super hot, and is perfect for those just beginning. It doesn't involve a whole lot of effort, and you can use this to get better acclimated to the sub and dom dynamic. If you're not used to giving or relinquishing control, this is the perfect activity, since it will help you get used to doing this, and getting a better feel for this.

Of course, you should always talk about what's cool and what's not cool before you begin. Even having the arms tied behind the woman's back while she does oral, it can be a fun thing. It's mostly just getting acclimated to the feeling, and the roleplay aspect of it can be really hot.

Pervertible

What in the world is that? Well, it's essentially a fancy word for various everyday objects that you have that can be used as toys. These include using canes, belts, rules, anything with a metal guide, spoons, brushes, or even little pieces of fur. These little pervertible are different things that you can use, and they're fun toys.

Now, I do suggest not inserting any of these toys. Foreign objects in orifices that don't belong there are only going to create problems. You should keep most of these to impact play, or just for sensation reasons, such as in the case of blindfolding someone and rubbing something soft or furry against the body for pleasure. You should definitely consider this, but use your discretion when choosing some toys.

Sensation play

Speaking of blindfolds, let's discuss sensation play! What is that? Essentially, it's restraining someone, or even yourself, blindfolding, and then putting sensations on the body. This can be anything from running something soft over their body, pinching and teasing to the edge, or even spanking. This is a very interesting one for both the dom and the sub.

The dom has complete control over you in this case, and the sub will surrender control. But, the cool thing about being blindfolded, is the fact that everything in essence gets heightened in terms of sensation. You'll feel various sensations that are much stronger than you would with your eyes open, and it can be a bit of a scary thing, but if you have trust in your partner know they're not going to completely mess you up, then you should be fine.

Flogging

Similar to spanking is flogging. Flogging is a bit of a step up from normal spanking, since it does look intense and scary, but it can be a bit of a shocking and pleasurable thing for a person. The pain isn't too much either. If you're looking to get into more pain play, use this don't bother getting a cane just yet, because caning is much more painful.

A flogger is good for all aspects of the body too, and a little bit goes a long way in terms of force.

Clothespins

And finally, we have clothespins. **Now,** it's important that, you start these on areas that aren't super sensitive. **For example,** don't put this on the clit or nipples first and foremost. That shit hurts. Instead, put it on the stomach, inner thigh, or any place that isn't too sensitive. From there, you can then move to other areas, and you can incorporate other activities into this, especially if you want to try this.

Now, you should always keep your partner's wishes at the forefront. You should always make sure that you know the limits, and respect them. But, these beginner activities are perfect for newbies, and if you've ever been curious, now is the time.

Chapter 8: Aftercare and Why You NEED It

So, you may have heard that after a session, you need some aftercare. What is that though? Why does it matter? Well, let's discuss some aftercare tips, tricks, and why you need this. The focus of this chapter is to get the reader to understand that aftercare is very important, and it's a focal part of a session.

What is it?

If you've seen 50 shades, you've probably literally seen Christian leave Anna, and that's a big NONO. The reason for this, is because after the height of the organ, the drop tends to happen.

Aftercare in essence is checking in with the person you just had a play session, or even a scene, happen, and you want to make sure they feel good about what happened to them. If there are bruises, the dom may bring some ice. If the woman is a bit shook up, the dom will take care of them, and in essence it involves giving them emotional care as well as physical care.

If there are injuries, you ALWAYS tend to them afterwards.

Remember, as we said before, BDSM releases endorphins. When you get smacked around, the pain sends a signal to the brain. Which will release endorphins. Those are the happy hormones, and you can get those practically overtaking your body.

Problem is, immediately after, the high of the orgasm causes a drop, and this can make people feel really bad. However, aftercare can help prevent the onslaught of shock after the session. Typically, it involves cuddling and conversation, since it is a time to help mellow out after the shock of a scene.

You may think that BDSM is just flogging and spanking, but it's not. While it is fun, you do need to incorporate some love and aftercare after what just went down.

You may wonder what makes BDSM different from actual abuse, violence, and coercion, and that is two things: consent, and aftercare. Consent is a huge part of it, as we discussed before, but aft care is just as important.

Aftercare can actually be a program too. When you've done this enough, your sub will know immediately what makes them feel good after the high of the orgasm. Oftentimes, the sub will enter something called subspace, which is altered psychological states that can happen when you have intense physical and mental stimulation, similar to being on a drug "high."

Aftercare, when done, will help the sub feel safer and they will feel appreciated after the sexual boundaries have been pushed. This is literally anything from being wrapped in a blanket, to even being made a sandwich after the shock of the situation.

Aftercare is important whether you've screwed your partner thousands of times, or even if you've never done this before. When the orgasms are finished, it's a way to feel good, since it essentially communicates "hey, thanks for letting me experience this very personal part of me."

So how do you do it?

With aftercare, it's a personal thing. But, the biggest thing to do, is to make sure the person is safe. It can be anything from driving the sub home so they're safe.

When starting out, or focusing on more vanilla sex, it's emotional more than physical. It doesn't have to be super sentimental, creative, or huge either, but in essence it's a display of acknowledging, humanity, and appreciation. For example, taking a shower together, cuddling, talk about how good the sex was, sharing a treat together, getting some water, helping them get themselves together, or even giving them a high five afterwards are perfect examples of aftercare, even in vanilla relationships.

Obviously, if you're going to be doing more forceful versions of BDSM, including impact play and the like, you need to make sure that you do a bit more on the physical side. But, that emotional comfort after all of that, doing what is said and done, can make a huge difference.

And it isn't even just in BDSM either. It's something that you should honestly do period after a good romp in the bedroom. You should use aftercare regardless really.

So, What ISN'T Aftercare

We've talked about what is, but what's isn't? Well, it's essentially not really making sure the other person is good after a session.

For example, sneaking out in the morning without saying goodbye, feeling ashamed or even aloof after that, feeling embarrassed after all of what you've done, or essentially treating the person as well, just body parts and refusing to acknowledge that you banged a person.

Essentially, this is something that can come off as very hurtful to the sub. After all, they relinquished control to you, so you should at least be pretty nice and not a total douche after all this. This goes for both men and women, focusing on the dub essentially leaving the partner.

You can have "emotionless" sex, which really isn't emotionless because it's impossible to have good sex without feeling good or any emotion. No-strings attached sex is still feeling emotions, even if it's just getting your urges out. When there's feeling, you need to have some sort of aftercare. As a rule, the higher that you fly, the softer your pad must be when you land. So, if you see that your partner just had the biggest, most amazing fucking orgasm ever, don't just toss them to the side and leave them to fend for themselves.

You know what you do instead? You invest a bit of time in aftercare. Investing in this via aftercare doesn't mean you're completely consenting to some relationship that you've solidified that you're with them for time immemorial. No, that means that if you do have a one-night stand, a fuck buddy, friends with benefits, you should still at least take care of them and make sure that they're good.

You may not know how to incorporate aftercare if they're someone that you're not familiar with, but, you should make sure that they're all good to go. You should ask them if they need anything, or if they're fine. Remember, sex is an adventure, and sometimes, it can be quite stimulating and shocking for the body as well.

Other Aftercare Ideas

Not sure about what you should do? Well, here are a few aftercare ideas that can help you.

Physical ideas:

- Removing the restraints and blindfolds

- Getting the partner something to eat and drink since blood sugar levels tend to be skewered
- Giving them a blanket or something warm
- Kissing or caressing any parts that are marked during play
- Giving affection in a quiet atmosphere
- Using an intimate massage with a warm massage oil
- Using a bath or shower with your partner

Emotional aftercare:

- Discussing how you both felt after the scene
- Discuss the good and bad, what can be improved
- Give the partner assurance about the kink, telling them that it isn't weird that they enjoyed
- Try to continue the conversation for a bit until you're both aware of negative feelings
- Discuss what can be improved in on the future

So, does everyone need it

Sometimes you occasionally get the partner that may prefer to be alone than to cuddle and kiss. However, negotiating aftercare is something that you should do before you begin. If you are beginning with experimenting, and don't know what the partner wants, you should always communicate with your partner and discuss anything that they like, or anything that they don't. You should also discuss feelings after a scene, so that you can make sure that you give your partner the correct aftercare that they desire.

As another aside, many assume that aftercare is something that doms do for subs. Yes, it's something that many who do in the dominant role, but sometimes the sub needs a little bit of help too. They do experience the drop as well, similarly from the actions at hand, and sometimes, they need the emotional connection with the sub as well, giving you a normal, loving, and affectionate feeling in their relationship.

Aftercare is very important, and there aren't any real guidelines to this, but you need to be open, attentive, and accepting to the needs of the other person, and you should make sure that everyone is happy and satisfied after a scene, so that nothing bad goes awry from this.

Chapter 9: BDSM Cautions

When you're working to have a good experience with BDSM, there are always some cautions that you should make sure you follow, in order to have a killer experience. Luckily, we can go over a few of the cautions that are present, and what you should know about before you get into this.

Know Your Dom Before You Begin

When choosing a dom, typically you can check many alternative dating websites, but when you do, you shouldn't run in right away and choose the first one you want.

Always, sit down and get to know him, and take your time. Have a good conversation, and when ready, meet up in a public place. This is a place where you can sit down and talk.

You should never rush into these. They're not something you should use as a hook up, because you could end up dead at worst.

If you talk to a dom, and they're immediately listing all of the expectations, you don't go with this dominants know and earn their position, and they need to build any trust, respect, communication, honesty, and consent on both ends, because remember, the sub has the power.

Check-ins

One thing that you will want to make sure that happens is a check-in. They're very important for intense play, and in essence it's the dom checking on the sub, making sure they're fine during play. The sub should respond, and tell them that you're more than just fine. If you notice that you're feeling numb, or that something is starting to bruise, or you're done with the flogging, actually say something.

Check-ins can be as simple as asking if the bottoms do know and remember the safe words, if they're still conscious, and if everything is good. You need to use these responsibly, and not every five seconds, and if the bottom is happy, then this looks good.

Also, use your own discretion. If you feel dizzy, say it. If your sub looks dizzy and weak, or they look like they're in too much pain, stop and get some light sugars into the sub to help this with the effects.

What About Gags?

We talked a lot about using safe words. They're super important, but what if you're gagged. What if you're deaf? Well, you may wonder what to do then, because a small gargling sound won't stop a person, but there is a way for you to communicate that you need to stop, or if you need a second.

Sometimes, people will put something on the ankles, or the wrists, and they will move it to make a sound, and that means to stop. It also can involve holding up fingers. Sometimes, you can also use the method of threes, which means either three grunts, or three shakes of the head. If they can do three, you should be good. If not, stop the scene.

On using floggers

Lots of people love floggers. They're good for playing, and some love the sensation, and flogging is a great way to really experiment with your sub or dom.

They can be scary, but often, they actually don't feel like how they look, and often, they're not painful at all.

However, you shouldn't get the cheap and stiff floggers that you see at sex toy shops or online. You'll touch it, and notice that the lashes on this are stiff, along with being thick, and the edges tend to not be rounded, which means they are painful and can injure you. a flogger that's good often has little lashes that are soft, and they won't injure you and, if you like the idea of being flogged, but you don't like pain, consider investing in a deerskin flogger, since those don't hurt at all.

On paddling and spanking

If you're into paddling and spanking, you need to watch where you hit. You should paddle, flog, or spank the butt, the thighs, or the upper back. Sometimes, you can flog the breasts, but you should stay away from the lower back, kidneys, and the neck, and you should never strike the neck or face with anything.

You should also try to avoid your knee and ankle joints, along with the elbow. It may not seem like much, but the thing is, if you're being hit there multiple times, it can actually damage them quite quickly. They're fragile. Remember as well, that the person when they're bent over has the muscles stretched in a long fashion, which means that they're more vulnerable, so you should make sure that the long muscles aren't extended if you're going to be doing this.

Candle Wax

Candle wax is great for sensation play, and is often encouraged, but, the wax isn't created equal. If you want to experiment in this fashion with this wax, you should get paraffin candles that are plain white, similar to the ones that you find that are considered "emergency" candles. There are specialty BDSM candles you can get as well.

Scented and colored ones contain something called plasticizers in them, and that can make it much hotter and could end up burning the skin.

You should avoid any candles that are all black, along with beeswax candles, since these tend to burn extremely hot.

This is a fun type of sensation play, but you have to be safe when doing this, that's for sure.

Bondage Safety

We talked a little bit about bondage safety beforehand, but now, we're going to go into it in a deeper fashion. This is probably one of the most important aspects of BDSM, because this can kill a person if don't incorrectly, especially when circulation is cut off.

As stated before, starting a light scene with some scarves, handcuffs, and the like might be a good thing. But, if you want to get serious with this, you should start investing. Most of the time, the best stuff to tie a partner up with, are some rope or some high-quality restraints.

The handcuffs tend to work at the start, but they can be tight, so it might be best to go with the fuzzy handcuffs.

Also, as a word of caution, lots of times nylons and those fake handcuffs can tighten during play struggles, and it's important to realize that you don't want to be too tight with these. If you want to use handcuffs for serious scenes, get some real handcuffs that are police grade. This is because they have a double lock mechanism, which means that when you struggle, they don't squeeze up. It also doesn't make it uncomfortable for the person. However, you should always know how to get out of these, and the mechanism behind it.

Now, bondage is fun, but for the sub, you should always be aware whenever you notice that you have tingly hands, numbness, or if you notice that your feet are cold, because that's a sign that circulation is being lost. You can also get some scissors and bring them over to release the person if it's something that you can cut.

Now, you should never constrict the throat with bondage. That's because it can cause a heart attack, or even death. You should when you're restraining is make sure that you've got the two finger rule in place, especially when collaring. You should be able to slip a couple fingers underneath the collar. And, you should never pull it hard enough that'll constrict the throat passage.

Also, never leave a restrained person alone.

Emotional Safety

Always make sure that you have emotional safety implemented. You should always discuss the health risks that you have before you start playing, and you should make sure you know your tools, and are safe. Safety is mostly physical, but there is the mental and emotional injuries that can come about too. You should be in touch with all your feelings that are happening.

There are instances where the sub thinks that the idea of a play session is perfect, but as soon as they get into the situation, they start to have emotional struggles.

It's something that you should recognize, and if it's too much, you should refrain from doing this until the head space is better for the individual.

More Paddle Concerns

If you're wondering if there are cautions that you should keep in mind, there are. With paddles, you should make sure not to hit with a strap edge, and with a paddle, you will need to make sure you're cautious of where you're hitting the body part. Some areas that don't have fat on them, such as the shins, are bad examples. That hurts.

But, even some of the fleshy areas are not good places, such as the kidneys, lower back, and the spinal column. Anything that doesn't have a muscle or fat padding is essentially bone, and hitting that isn't good or safe. You should make sure that you discuss with your sub where you want to hit the person.

Sometimes, you need to have a diagram for this. Some people are fine with various areas, and not with others. Always have the discussion with the sub before you begin, and any health problems or sensitive body areas.

A heady paddle is often something that is discussed because when it does hit the backside, it's much different. If you're going to use a heavy paddle, you hit areas with more flesh on them. If you want to hit the lighter padded areas, you get a ruler. Also, if a person is stretched out when you're paddling, you should watch out for the sciatic nerve being stretched, because this leads to extremely bad pain, and can even lead to sciatica, which will leave someone out of commission for a long while.

Now, you can use a paddle in front, but only with a percussion to it that's lighter. Sometimes, some like the paddling of the breasts, but some doctors say this could lead to an increase in fibroids in women. This can cause a false positive when getting a mammogram. You can also do percussive play near where the genitalia are, but you also need to take precautions to it. Some like it, some hate it, but if they want it, you need to be very careful, and often, it's best to stick near the inner thighs, so definitely be gentle.

Paddles are often better to start off with than straps, since the paddles can be predictive on where they hit, and they are easy to target, so you won't be able to hurt someone.

If you get a paddle with holes, it'll be more severe, since there is less resistance to the air, and a decrease in the mass of it, which makes it easier to move. It will also give a smaller surface area, which means that if you do this, make sure that you do take your time to ensure your sub is cool with this.

Breath play Cautions

When you're using breath play, you should always make sure you know how to do it. It can cause permanent damage to the carotid arteries, which leads to numbness, dizziness, difficulties speaking, and weakness.

The larynx is very fragile, and easily touched. Pressure should be avoided, and any injury can lead to possible choking, inability to speak, or even the inability to breathe, so avoid this at all costs.

When choking, the airway can be obstructed by the tongue, and you might notice swelling of the lips and tongues, so it's impossible to tell just how much is happening, since everyone is different.

The reduction of the blood flow during this can also cause ischemia, which means that it's a reduction of oxygen to the brain, and hypoglycemia, which can cause a stroke, transient, brain infarction, brain edema, and other issues.

With this, it's best if you make sure that you have someone that knows what the heck they're doing. It has so many risks with it, and it does come with some questionable risks that can really affect the person. It's best that, if you do want to get into this, you seek out someone who knows exactly what they're doing, and knows how to attend to the risks involved.

With ball gags as well, there is some danger to it. If a person chokes on their vomit, unable to expel this, it actually goes into their lungs completely, and while this normally wouldn't draw completely into their lungs, the chances of this increases a lot. If the barrier is removed, it will not prevent the damage to the respiratory areas. This can lead to going unconscious, cyanosis, cardiac arrest, and also you may stop breathing.

You should also realize that if tape is used, there is also the risk of allergic reaction, which may cause swelling of areas, unconsciousness, potentially death in some cases, especially if they're allergic to the materials.

You should be very careful with any of this, and you should make sure that if you are going to take the risks, you do your research to ensure that you're safe.

When Meeting a Dom or Sub

It's also important to highlight the element of stranger danger, especially when choosing a new dom or sub. The thing is, if you've never met the person before, you're putting yourself at an insane risk. We did discuss the safety calls that you can use beforehand, but let's take a moment to talk about some tips when it comes to meeting the dom, or the sub.

First thing's first, actually have a conversation with them. Really get to know them. This person has to be someone that you trust, and if you don't fully trust them, that puts you at risk. Get to know each of them, and make sure that you're able to really connect.

If they're someone you met at a munch, you've probably already met them in person and had a great conversation. If not, and they're someone that you met over the internet, always, ALWAYS meet these people in a public place. Never meet them at a private residence, because the person may be a serial killer for all you know. Of course, that's a bit of an extreme, but the truth is, you don't fully know the person.

If you're not comfortable with meeting someone the first time, bring a friend. There is nothing wrong with that. You can also do the safety call here too.

If you notice that he's demanding a lot out of you immediately if it's a dom, then chances are this person isn't going to cater to the sub's needs, so make sure that you watch for this, and don't give in.

On the flip side, if the sub seems to be someone that has demands that you can't meet, you don't have to go into a contract with them. The thing with BDSM, is that you need to find someone that goes with your own sexual desires. You shouldn't just pick the first sub or dom that you see. That runs a lot of risks.

Also, for any sub, you need to remember to keep your heart in check. This person may eventually become someone as special as a lover to you, but that may not happen. You may never fall in love or get married to this person. Hell, this person may just be a sexual outlet. Some people do have doms that they go to for release, when they can't get it from a partner. That's something that some people like, and that's really their call. But if the relationship is strictly on a sexual plane, keep your heart out of this.

But of course, these cautions are all laid out. The best thing to do is to make sure that you take these precautions, and know exactly what you're doing, so that you can prevent an accident from happening.

Now, let's talk about some BDSM tips to help make your time with your sub or dom so much better. There is a lot that you can do here, and we're going to talk about them.

Start out slow

If you have a steady partner already, and you want to explore this, you can start with a couple of simple things.

This can be as simple as demanding your partner to go down on you, perhaps grabbing them by the hair and doing so, and you say they have to do it until you say you're done. You want to start trying to demand, and maybe start to see if the person likes it. If they do, then you can start getting a bit friskier with this.

Communicate like you Need To

Let's talk about communication. If you're not talking with your partner like your life depends on it, then you're going to have issues here. Sometimes, people get flustered in the heat of the moment, but you need to be communicative and trustworthy with your partner. It makes your life way easier.

With that being said, you should learn how to open up. BDSM is a personal thing, it caters to your desires, and there isn't one cookie cutter relationship out there. You don't have to get into BDSM scenes like those that you see in porn. You can do something light. You can release your expectations and cut loose if you feel like you're ready for that.

This also involves saying what you want. If you really want something, you say it. If you don't want something, bust out the safe word. You want something that's clear, since it will help you make sure that your boundaries are established, and that misunderstandings don't occur.

Start with Some Sex Toys

If you've ever wanted to try sex toys, but you haven't, now is the time. You can try out BDSM toys such as clamps. Clamps are usually really good, but you should try it yourself and see if you like it. You can even try squeezing to see if they like it. Trying out new sexual toys can give you that new and fuzzy feeling of trying to understand, and it'll allow you to get a better feel for whatever you're going into.

Try getting curious

One thing to try is getting curious. Lots of people, if they've never tried BDSM before, start to grow curious. Maybe they're utterly sick of their vanilla sex life and want something new, or maybe they've always had these feelings, but didn't know how to approach them. If that's the case, then you should learn to embrace it. BDSM involves a lot of sexual curiosity. You should, if you've been curious about something, become inclined to try it. The worst that you can say is you dislike it, and tell your partners to stop.

Another thing that can really come into play here, is becoming a voyeur. The idea of watching other people have sex might be a bit weird, but you can learn to start embracing sex, being comfortable with it, and getting curious about new ideas from watching. Some people think that it's a negative thing, but it's something that's been hardwired into a lot of us, which means that negative notions need to have healthier ones put in. You can go to sex parties, which are common when getting into BDSM, and you'll see others going at it, without you having to perform. There's a little voyeur in everyone, and this could end up being something that you may enjoy.

All in all, learn to get kinky. You should start to learn to explore, and lots of times, BDSM doesn't even involve genitalia sex, so it's okay to get curious, use the imagination, and have a little bit of fun.

Trust is Necessary

This is something you should know by now, but trust isn't something that's automatically given. You need to give yourself some time. This is something that you need to actually make sure that is put in before you decide to start or even continue a true D/s relationship. This takes a lot of time, consider ion, and energy as well. You should start off with a slow build, and don't start with just showing up and demanding to whip your partner. That's not how you do it. This is a huge trust thing, and often, if there isn't enough trust there, you're going to end up creating a lot of upset between yourself, and your partner. So be smart, and wait a bit.

Own up to mistakes

If a dom fucks up in some way, that's breaking consent. That's a serious thing that can happen, and it's important to admit when you've totally screwed up. The dom needs to realize this, and be honest about this. If there was a breach of consent, you need to own up to it, and the sub shouldn't be quiet about it either. If there is a dom that ends up screwing up, they need to own up to their mistakes, and learn from this, and for the sub, it's okay if you do speak up on it. Lots of times, if the sub is honest about it, and the dom cares more about telling others than the reputation, lots of doms are more respected in that regard.

Talk afterwards

If you talk about the scene afterwards, it can help with the relationship. This is important because the body language that you have does indicate whether or not someone is having a good time. However, with BDSM, it's a little more complicated. Lots of times, someone might like the feeling of being slapped around, with tears coming out of their eyes and a look of pain on their face. You may wonder if you should stop, but they're enjoying this. However, after the scene is over, sit down and talk about this, because it will tell you what they liked, and what they didn't appreciate, so you can fix the scene up afterwards.

Wear to feel Good

Lots of times, people think you have to wear all this leather or pleather, but that's not the case. BDMS doesn't have to be that, but if you're looking to really get a lot of fun out of this, wear what will make you feel empowered. Got a sexy and sleek red dress that you know hugs your curves and makes you feel good? Well, wear that.

Teasing

One way to really get your partner going is to tease them for a little bit. You can start to talk about getting a few things, and demanding that the other doesn't put it on, but if they do it's at their own risk. You can even get chastity devices put on your partner, meaning they can't have sex for a couple of days. It's a bit of a bigger thing, but sometimes, the tease is something that others enjoy.

Pictures

With BDSM, it's a bit of a very private activity. Unless the person consents to sending pictures, then don't send them. You don't need to prove this, and the real-life rules are still a thing.

Power play Outside of Sex

Not into totally getting into power play yet? Well, why not try power play outside of sex? This can be involving ordering the food that your partner has, telling them the outfit that they will wear, or even giving them rules for the evening or day, and if they do end up breaking them, they get punished each time. It's quite interesting, and it's something that you can try out.

Don't Be Goal Oriented

One thing that you do need to not do, is starting to demand goals out of people. Don't treat sex as a sort of goal, but rather it's a journey. When you are doing this, don't talk about the acts that you're doing, and the specific acts, you should talk as well about how you feel.

Lots of times, people put in the base system where the home run is only intercourse with the penis and vagina. Rather than thinking that sex is something that eventually results in that, you should start to explore in other ways. Stop always having the same goals, and make a few changes for yourself.

You should always take baby sets, and make sure that you start with something that's small, and from there continue on. Baby steps are the way to do it, and the way to be successful.

Stop the Stereotype

Not every single dom is a sociopath, and not every single sub has mom and dad issues, but rather everyone is different. You should make sure that it's okay for a man to be submissive, and that it doesn't make him weak. Sometimes, people are fine with being a submissive, because it means that he trusts you. Even the biggest alphas can end up being submissive in the bedroom, and it's something that you just need to curb.

All assumptions should be left at the door. It's about your own personal little desires, and it's important to start to understand, and cater to this different sort of lifestyle.

Conclusion

As you can see here, BDSM is way more than just whips and chains, but rather, it's about communication, trust, and consent of sexual practices done in the safest manner possible. There is a lot here, and it might be a lot to take in.

Sometimes, the best way to get experience is to go to a BDSM munch, or even a local dungeon, and learn from there. There are doms and subs that are out there that can help you. If you want a professional dom or domme, you should seek them out, and find out just what you want from it, and see if this works.

Some people like this type of sexual play. It's something that you can try with your partner, take baby steps, and learn to enjoy. Remember, you don't have to be completely restrained when you do this, but instead, become open and willing to try new things, and from there, make the best that you can out of this, and make it so that you're happy with the way things are.

With that being said, your next step is to figure out what you want from a BDSM relationship, and what you think works for you. It's a very personal thing, and something that you can enjoy, so do it at your own enjoyment, and choose what you want to do. Start to get used to this, and you'll be shocked at the difference it makes in your life.

Made in United States
Troutdale, OR
11/26/2023

14902513R00046